Get Well Soon

Dr KEITH M. SOUTER
DSc, MB, CHB, MRCGP, MHMA

Get Well Soon

NATURAL REMEDIES TO AID CONVALESCENCE
FROM ILLNESS, BIRTH, TRAUMA AND SURGERY

Index compiled by Barbara Newby

SAFFRON WALDEN
THE C.W.DANIEL COMPANY LIMITED

First published in Great Britain in 1996
by The C.W.Daniel Company Limited
1 Church Path, Saffron Walden
Essex, CB10 1JP, England

© Keith M. Souter 1996

ISBN 0 85207 297 X

This book is printed on part-recycled paper

Produced in association with
Book Production Consultants plc Cambridge
Typeset by Cambridge Photosetting Services
Printed and bound by St. Edmundsbury Press,
Bury St. Edmunds, Suffolk.

*For my brothers George and John,
and in memory of our late father John Snr.
Together we were an unbeatable team.*

CONTENTS

INTRODUCTION

No-one can doubt the advances of modern Medicine. Drugs have become more powerful, more specific, more readily available. Similarly, surgery has also taken a leap forward. Organ transplantation, keyhole surgery and microsurgical techniques have brought relief to millions.

Yet just as the treatments have become better, so too have social forces become more acute. Since treatments are perceived as being swift and effective there is an expectation placed upon people that they should return to 'normal' activities as quickly as possible. No longer do people have the time to convalesce back to health.

The problem is that the human body needs time to recover. Undue pressures often only complicate recovery by reducing overall resistance and producing a tendency to relapse or develop complications. It is, perhaps, for this reason that we see so many more problems of immunity, so many more cases of stress-related illness, and so many more cases of Chronic Fatigue and ME.

After two decades of medical practice I have come to the conclusion that we almost have to view convalescence as a separate stage from the actual health event from which one is recovering. It is a time when the individual needs to take active steps to aid recovery to normal health, rather than just accept the usual advice about time, good food and a little rest.

This little book is not meant to replace medical advice, but to complement it. It looks at natural strategies and supplements which can be taken during convalescence in order to *Get Well Soon.*

Keith Souter

CHAPTER 1

CONVALESCENCE AFTER THE EVENT

Patients may recover in spite of drugs or because of them.
Gaddum, 1959

The silver-haired doctor removed his stethoscope and coiled it before dropping it into his old-fashioned black gladstone bag. Then he smiled as he looked down at me. I was lying in bed, feeling completely drained of energy. The old doctor had visited me three times in the previous week.

"You've had a particularly bad case, you know. It's sapped your reserves, so you'll have to give yourself time to convalesce."

He ticked off a number of points on his fingers as he explained just what I should and shouldn't do during my recovery time.

"Follow my advice and you'll be raring to go in a fortnight," he said as he picked up his bag and made for the door. "Ignore it and you'll be back to square one in no time at all."

I was a fresh young medical student and I was anxious to get back to my studies. I had important exams looming and I thought that I simply couldn't afford to take time off. But as it was, I soon realised the wisdom of his words. I heeded his advice and put my studies out of my head until I was able to resume them with a clear head and renewed stamina.

I still feel that if it had not been for his advice I may have fared less favourably in my meeting with the examiners some little time later. But the most important thing that I learned, the thing that I am most grateful to that doctor for, was the insight he gave me into the need to convalesce.

Convalescence, from the Latin *con*, and *valescere*, meaning 'to grow strong', is a concept that people pay lip-service to these days. Powerful drugs are seen to

1

'kill off' disease, keyhole surgery allows the removal of organs in an increasingly less invasive manner, and there is now a trend to mobilise new mothers almost immediately after childbirth. The old idea that you need to convalesce after a major event is becoming redundant as people are being encouraged to resume work as swiftly as possible. Unfortunately, many will not have convalesced properly, they will return to their daily life still feeling less than well, still being at risk of having another illness event.

The fact is that the main focus of practical Medicine is on treatment of *the event.* From their earliest days in medical school, doctors are taught that the all-important thing is the diagnosis.

This labelling allows the doctor to imagine how the pathological process is affecting the individual's tissues, his metabolic processes, and which ultimately produces symptoms and signs of the disease. Having then arrived at the diagnosis, a suitable treatment is initiated in the fond hope and belief that it will eventually return the patient to health.

So entrenched in us nowadays is the idea of illness and disease as enemies, that we talk of drugs as being *magic bullets*, and of therapies as belonging to some *therapeutic armoury.* Now I am not going to decry modern drugs. As a conventionally trained doctor I am only too well aware of the life-saving and life-improving nature of many of these drugs, as well as the magnificent advances of modern surgery. What I am suggesting is that wonderful though these treatments may be, they do not provide the whole answer. They do not in themselves bring about the recovery towards health. It is the body's own recuperative ability that does so.

There is a view, adopted and practised by many health workers, that the treatment of the event is all that is necessary. The treatment is seen as setting the individual's metabolism, energy network, or however one cares to think of it, back on track. It is then considered just a matter of time before the recovery takes place.

2

Actual observation, however, shows that it is just not so simple. People recover at different rates and in different ways. Indeed, as we shall see in the next chapter, there are many recovery patterns which have to be taken into account. Some people will recover smoothly and swiftly, while others may be plagued by complications, relapse and a very slow convalescence.

HEALTH AND ILLNESS

The World Health Organisation's definition of health is *'a state of complete physical, mental and social well-being and not just the absence of disease and infirmity.'*

It is not a bad definition, but it is a difficult one to apply. When you think about it, many people would be hard put to feel well in all three areas all the time. Indeed, an international study in the early 1970s revealed that only 10 per cent of the population would consider themselves well according to the WHO criteria. A similar 10 per cent would consider themselves to be in poor health. Of the remaining 80 per cent, half would consider themselves to be in good health although not in all three areas and half would consider themselves to be in only fair health.

Another contemporary study revealed that one could expect 60 per cent of the population to be taking medication of some sort on any one day. Of that total, half would be taking a prescribed treatment and half would be self-medicating with some treatment or tonic. They would either be treating themselves for the event or trying to get better afterwards.

There is obviously a spectrum of well-being. Some people perceive themselves to be ill when others would not. It seems that individual coping mechanisms have a lot to do with it.

Essentially, a coping mechanism is some means of modifying a stress so that it doesn't actually produce strain. Take for example the case of a man who is under continual harassment from both his boss and his customers when he is at work. He cannot argue with the boss and he cannot afford to upset the

3

customers, so he waits until the end of the day and he chops logs. He is coping by sublimating his anger and frustration to the logs. Or take the case of a woman who deals with her chronic pain by always remembering that her mother had a far worse problem than she has.

These are both simplistic examples, but they serve to illustrate the point. Some people are good at developing or acquiring coping mechanisms. Some people adopt a philosophical approach to their life and to the hardships they have to endure. Others may feel the pressure at the first sign of adversity and be unable to cope with illness or trauma.

EVENTS AFFECTING WELL-BEING

The feeling of health is never constant. We are all aware of fluctuations in our well-being, pretty well in keeping with our physical, mental and social state. At times we feel physically unwell, at times our emotional equanimity is affected by happenings in our lives, and at other times we are affected by problems in our actual environment.

In this book I refer to an *event* as the point at which one loses that sense of well-being and feels ill. It is the time when some form of healing is taking place. There are several types of health-event that ought to be considered:

ILLNESS

Here we refer to actual pathological states arising from some disease process. There are, of course, several disease patterns that have different significances.

Acute Minor Events – these are the minor coughs, colds, gastric upsets and other minor ailments. They are conditions which the body will throw off in good time, generally without any intervention from a doctor.

Acute Intermediate Events – these are the severe, ultimately curable conditions, such as prolonged chest infections, pneumonias, etc. Those conditions in which the individual may have been totally unable to do any of their simple daily tasks for a matter of a fortnight or more.

4

Acute Major Events – these are the more serious conditions such as heart attacks and strokes. Medical treatment is necessary as an emergency to prevent possible fatality. They are almost inevitably going to create fears about the individual's future mortality, and about the chance of having another more serious event at a later date.

Chronic Events – these are ongoing health problems from one condition. This is the Rheumatoid Arthritis, the Chronic Bronchitis type of problem. They are difficult because of the continuous treatment that seems to be needed, and because there may be a tendency to deteriorate.

TRAUMA

Sudden unexpected alterations in one's well-being through accidents or violence create emotional shock and physical discomfort. There may be a fear of not improving to the previous level of fitness or function. Also, there may be persisting emotional trauma secondary to the shock of the original problem.

Broken bones bring frustration, since they clearly affect one's physical well-being in terms of functional ability, yet do not necessarily cause pain after the acute part of the trauma is over.

CHILDBIRTH

There is no other event that can be so satisfying for a woman than to produce a child. But there is a profound physiological change to be gone through at the same time. One's circulation changes dramatically, the hormone levels drop suddenly, the whole inner structure of one's abdomen and pelvis changes in the course of a few days.

A few decades ago women were more or less forced to take time to lie-in, or convalesce. Now there is no time given, even after the combined event which some women have to go through when they give birth by Caesarian Section.

Virtually every mother experiences some upset in their mood in the first few days and weeks. A new person has been born, bringing with them new responsibilities, new demands. There can be feelings of depression, irritability, inadequacy or even guilt. These all have to be resolved and healed, just as much as any physical wound would.

EMOTIONAL TRAUMAS

These, like physical illness, can take acute or chronic forms. They need healing and understanding. They can be exhausting mentally and physically. Indeed, when the emotions are strained, one's resistance is lowered so that some other problem can seem insurmountable.

TREATMENT

Finally, one cannot discount the effects of the treatment itself. This will be cumulative to the other event involved, but sometimes it can be a significant feature in itself.

Surgery has a variable effect, depending upon whether it was major or minor surgery, whether done under a local or a general anaesthetic, and whether the surgery was curative (eg for appendicitis) or palliative (eg a drainage operation for an inoperable cancer); mutilating (eg a mastectomy for cancer of the breast) or cosmetic (eg a face-lift or breast augmentation). The mental state of the individual may have just as much a part to play in convalescence as the actual physical healing.

Radiotherapy and chemotherapy for malignant conditions both create potential problems. They can both produce physical symptoms, such as pain and nausea, and they are both subject to the same anxieties that accompany surgery for serious conditions. If they are done in patients who have also had such surgery then the effects can be cumulative.

Medical treatment with drugs can also create several problems. There may be after-effects upon the bowel with antibiotics, rebound phenomena with steroids, and persisting nausea, tiredness and headaches with various heart and respiratory drugs.

6

HEALING MECHANISMS

The body is constantly striving to keep itself in a state of good repair. This is no mean feat since in the average adult body there are between 75 and 100 million million cells. These fall into about 100 different types which are arranged into specialised groups to form tissues. In turn these are organised into organs which function with others to produce organ systems. Each system fulfils a set of functions, yet is interdependent upon the other functioning systems of the body.

Homoeostasis is the name given to the overall process whereby the body maintains its internal functioning. It includes the maintenance of the body fluid balance, the control of temperature, metabolism and the overall maintenance of the number of cells within the tissues.

The turnover of cells within the systems varies greatly. This is inevitable, since some systems have greater demands laid upon them. The more specialised the function of the cell, however, the longer it has to last.

In Medicine, the cells are grouped into three categories according to the ease with which they can regenerate. First of all there are the *labile* cells which are continually being replaced throughout life. Skin cells and the lining cells of the respiratory system, the bowel, bone marrow and lymph glands are all examples.

Secondly there are the *stable* cells which usually stop multiplying in early adult life. That is, they have a slow turnover for the rest of the individual's life, unless called upon to regenerate because of illness or injury. The cells of the liver, pancreas, thyroid, kidneys and adrenal glands are all examples.

Finally, there are the *permanent* cells which are virtually incapable of regeneration after birth. Injury to these tissues can be catastrophic. The voluntary muscles and the cells of the central nervous system are examples of these highly specialised cells.

Whenever a tissue is strained or injured, the normal reparative processes that maintain the numbers of cells at an optimum start to work overtime. The process of *inflammation* is an integral part of this activity.

ACUTE INFLAMMATION – People generally think of inflammation as being a bad thing. In fact, the presence of inflammation indicates that the body is try-ing to heal itself. The characteristic components of an inflammatory process are redness, heat and swelling. The redness and heat are due to dilation of local blood vessels, the aim being to divert more blood to the area to bring oxygen, nutrients and repair cells, and to carry away metabolites.

The swelling is produced by the leakage of fluid from the small blood vessels. With this fluid white blood cells start mopping up invading organisms (if any) and cellular debris. Sometimes the numbers of white cells will be so great that pus is formed. At this stage pain is liable to occur because of stretching and irritation of the tissues and penetrating nerves.

Once the acute episode is over, the next phase of new cell production to replace the others takes place. If the wound or area is clean and the process has been performed well, then the regeneration may take place fairly uneventfully. This is most likely where the cell loss has been mainly of *labile* cells. If the physical structure has been affected, however, or if the area of the body contains a large number of *stable* or *permanent* cells then the healing is liable to involve a lot of scar formation. This obviously is functionally less effective than the regeneration of the original cell types.

CHRONIC INFLAMMATION – often the factor producing the stress and strain upon the organ or tissue is of a milder but more persistent nature. When this happens the redness, heat and swelling may not be so obvious, yet the inflammatory process persists. Excess scar tissue is formed and the normal structure of the organ or tissue becomes deranged and func-tionally less and less effective. The chronic inflamma-tion seen in conditions like Rheumatoid Arthritis, various liver and respiratory diseases are examples.

In chronic inflammatory conditions the pain may be

quite different from that of acute inflammatory conditions. It no longer serves a useful function in that it warns about a problem. It merely grinds on and can be extremely disabling.

NECROSIS – this is the name given to the death of cells and tissue; the result of degeneration of the cells. It can be thought of as the end point, after a cell under strain finally swells, becomes functionless and therefore dies. The changes of necrosis reduce it to a form in which it can be removed by the inflammatory cells.

CONVALESCENCE

The recovery, or convalescent state, includes the continuation of the physical reparative process plus the general increase in resistance, strength and emotional status necessary for the individual to obtain once again that feeling of well-being.

As we shall see in the next chapter, the recovery pattern is dependent upon many variables. While it may be that many people will just get better given tender loving care (TLC), rest and good food, others may need more than that.

Over the last few decades we have seen a rise in the number of people with Chronic Fatigue Syndrome, also known under several other names, such as Yuppie Flu and ME. Although this is rather a blanket description for a number of differing problems, it is likely that for one reason or another the individual simply did not convalesce or recover properly. What should have been a normal recovery developed into a chronic fatigue state.

My contention is that convalescence is actually a separate state on its own. Like the actual event which causes the illness or *dis-ease*, it can be ameliorated or improved by the use of appropriate remedies. Very often, however, one of the main brakes upon the individual's recovery is the fact that they still suffer from the after-effects of the *event-treatment*. This too may need to be taken into account. In my view, since recovery is a natural process, the best remedies to aid that recovery are natural ones.

CHAPTER 2

RECOVERY PATTERNS

Thou cunning'st pattern of excelling nature....
William Shakespeare, *Othello*

The physician should practise the Art of prognosis
Hippocrates

After an illness or significant life or health event, patients are often told that they can expect to get better in so many days, so many weeks, so many months. The expectation is that they will improve in a linear straightforward pattern. This rarely happens. There are various ways that people recover. Some people know that they are slow healers, or fast healers. Some are impatient, others are stoical, and so on. But before we talk about recovery patterns, what is recovery?

To most people it means a return to their normal level of health. To some it may be an improvement in their general health, because a diseased part has been removed surgically, an abscess has resolved, or an inflamed organ has reverted to its non-inflamed state. To many others the recovery may be to a lesser level than their previous state of 'normality'.

There is an important point to make here, because people often imagine that their current state of health is independent of the past. This is not the case at all, since we are today fashioned from all that has happened to us throughout our lives. Every illness, every experience, forgotten or remembered, will have exerted some influence in making the individual the person he is today.

DYNAMIC CREATURES
It is usually assumed that an individual's past medical history stretches out behind him in a linear fashion,

with illness or health events being designated as milestones along the old trail of his life. As such, it is thought that most of those past events will have been burned out and have no relevance other than as medical historical details.

This idea of linearity is actually the way that most of us think in the West. It is a medical model which is very limited, however. While it accepts that the loss of a limb will affect one's mobility, or the loss of an organ will affect one's physiological functioning, it pays little regard to the effect of a past bereavement, a bad attack of glandular fever in adolescence, or a severe dose of measles in childhood.

Most people involved in health care will have observed that at times past conditions flare up. They will experience past physical and psychological reactions. And often those reactions will appear during the course of the illness or in the recovery from it.

The reason for this is that human beings are dynamic creatures. We are not static in any sense. Like the rest of the matter which makes up the physical universe, we are composed of atoms and molecules. Hugely complicated arrangements of molecules make up the building bricks of living cells. And as stated in Chapter one, in the average adult body there are between 75 and 100 million million cells which are arranged into tissues and ultimately into organs and organ systems.

We also know from the new physics that all matter is vibrational. That is, at any moment in time, a subatomic particle can behave and exist as either particulate matter or as a form of energy. Essentially, this means that our perception of ourselves as existing in a physical universe is simply a result of the limitation of our senses. The reality is that we are vibrational. As such, every experience of the individual's life is part of that vibrational pattern.

In terms of the medical history, think of it as being like the layers of a pearl or the layers of an onion. Each health event is a layer. As the body copes with the particular problem, it gets walled off, seemingly limiting it to the past. The reality, however, is that the vestige of the event continues to exert an effect, in that it still contributes to the overall vibrational pattern of the individual. It may no longer exert any obvious effect because the body has coped with it. Nevertheless, it is still there, possibly awaiting release, or acting as a brake to subsequent recovery from some other problem.

Figure 1 shows a representation of a vibrational pattern in which the different layers represent past illnesses. The shells show the effects of seemingly walled-off episodes of measles, asthma and eczema.

Figure 2 shows the situation when someone is suffering from their eczema. The outermost shell is active.

Figure 3 shows a common finding when the above individual has their eczema treated. The outer layer is effectively dispersed, allowing the inner shell to become active as a flare up of asthma.

This is a very simple example of the vibrational model of health. Any of the underlying layers may be affected if exposed by something occurring in the outer layers, or if something happens to directly stimulate the lower layers themselves.

Trauma is one type of stimulus that can cause a flare-up of some past problem. For example, if someone has a history of kidney troubles in childhood, then receives a blow to the back over the kidney area as an adult, the kidney problem can flare-up again.

Similarly, if a past inflammatory condition has seemingly burned itself out, it can be flared up if another apparently unrelated condition causes a diminution in resistance of the body. In this case it may be that the body's resistance was holding the past problem in check, keeping the problem 'walled-off' as an inactive layer (Figure 4). The new or current condition then removes the resistance allowing the underlying past problem to flare up (Figure 5).

The effect of activation of past problem layers can account for much of the unpredictability of health. The activated layer may manifest itself as a flare-up of a past health problem, or exert an effect on the

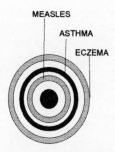

FIGURE 1 All conditions walled off

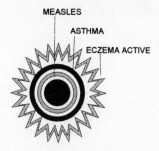

FIGURE 2 Active eczema

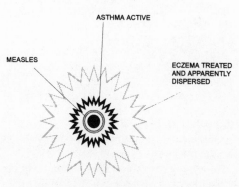

FIGURE 3 Treated eczema followed by flare-up
of asthma

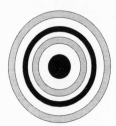

FIGURE 4 Walled-off episodes, no problems

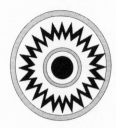

FIGURE 5 Lowered resistance causing flare-up of past problem

current state of health. This may, of course, be through a complicated chain reaction occurring through the interaction of several layers. This may hamper recovery, produce a complication, or cause a relapse (Figure 6).

FIGURE 6 Flare-ups and chain reaction causing relapse or complications

RECOVERY PATTERNS
As I mentioned at the start of this chapter, there are various ways in which one can recover from a life or health event. If you look at Figure 7 as you read this section, you will probably recognise patterns that either yourself, a friend, relative or patient has experienced.

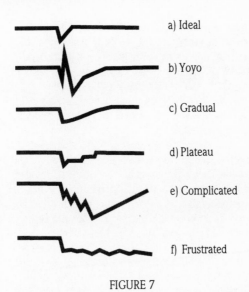

FIGURE 7

1) The ideal recovery – the health event causes a short illness followed by a swift and unimpeded return to usual normal health. This is the typical response in a young healthy individual to a simple self-limiting viral illness.

2) The yoyo recovery phenomenon – the health event is initially short-lived, followed by a fast recovery – perhaps too fast – to a state of euphoria and enhanced energy. This state does not last long, but is followed by a complete relapse and a subsequent slow recovery. This is often the case in psychological problems or when there is much psychological stress. The stress may come from subtle pressures to recover quickly.

3) The gradual upward recovery – after a major health event (indicated by the depth of the event spike), such as a non-fatal heart attack, pneumonia or non-complicated trauma, the recovery takes time, but is usually complete to previous health, or an acceptable limited level.

4) The plateau recovery – after the event the individual recovers quickly to a level at which they

15

plateau. This often produces frustration and anxiety, since the individual will inevitably wonder why they are not recovering in a straight linear fashion. Usually, there will be a series of plateaus, each to a level of recovery higher than the one before. This is the common recovery after an uncomplicated surgical operation, where a diseased part has been successfully completely removed.

5) *The complicated recovery* – after the event the individual's recovery is marred by at least one complication. Each one impairs the resistance and recovery components of homoeostasis, permitting a further complication to occur. Thus the individual has not only to get over the original event, but also get over each complication. The deep vein thrombosis after an operation or period of immobilization is a good example of this, since other complications can follow.

6) *The frustrated recovery* – here the individual never achieves a proper recovery, since the first illness or event so depletes the reserves that he sustains a succession of minor illnesses. These seem to be trivial in themselves, but their effect is to keep the individual's reserves in a depleted state so that very little recovery actually takes place. Often antibiotics or other suppressant treatment will have been given for many of these secondary illnesses or events, so that the body's own healing mechanisms are never allowed to function properly. Also, trying to rush back to health without adequate convalescence seems common. This may well be the natural history of Chronic Fatigue Syndrome, also known by the name of Myalgic Encephalomyelitis or ME.

CONSTITUTIONAL TYPES

Each person is unique. Although two people may have exactly the same medical history, having had the same infections, the same immunisations and a similar history of trauma, yet they will probably respond to their illnesses in different ways. One may be forced to bed with the slightest cold, while the other always feels better if they keep on the move. You will probably have noticed this among your own family and friends. Some people have hardier constitutions than others.

This observation is one of the basic principles of Homoeopathy and other natural therapies. Each person has a constitutional type which will broadly modify the response to an illness or health event. For example, someone who always has to take to bed with a respiratory infection is unlikely to be helped by being forced to get out into the open air and soldier on. On the other hand, the type who is better for being up and about will not thrive when they are forced to rest in bed.

The constitution encompasses much more than illness response. It includes the general outlook of the individual, their likes and dislikes, their predispositions to physical and emotional stress, and such things as their appearance.

Returning to Figures 1–6, notice that there is a kernel, a core represented in each diagram. This is the constitutional type; the very essence of the individual which will modify the whole vibrational pattern.

In convalescence from an illness or health event one should try to listen to the body, to obey the nature of one's constitutional type. It is quite wrong for everyone to adopt the same recovery plan, since some convalescent regimes will be directly opposed to the recovery needs of some individuals' constitutions. Admittedly, this is not always an easy matter, since many people never really look deeply at themselves. Indeed, in today's society people often strive to imitate favourite role models. Unfortunately, the role model they adopt may also be far from appropriate.

As a start I believe that one cannot do better than look at one's dominant mental thought process. Look at the main negative mental symptoms that one experiences. Know this and you are a long way along the path to getting yourself better. We will return to this in the next chapter.

17

THE NEED TO CONVALESCE

In days gone by people used to take time to recover, to convalesce after an illness, a childbirth, operation or injury. Nowadays people are persuaded that because of medical advances the treatment one receives is automatically better. Not only that, but because of financial and occupational pressures, people are actively encouraged to resume work or activity as swiftly as possible.

As a conventionally trained doctor I accept that modern treatments have done much to improve the actual weathering of the storm. They have helped to shorten the actual illness or health event. But they have done little to help the recovery process afterwards. I ask you to again consider Figure 2, showing the situation when someone is experiencing the actual current illness. Modern treatments are good at limiting this, but they do not tackle the situation in Figures 3, 5 and 6. In other words they merely attack the main presenting problem, but not the other problems that are contributing to it from the past.

I believe that recovery or convalescence is a separate stage from the illness itself. The actual recovery to optimum health occurs when the vibrational pattern reaches a stage of neutrality where the past problems cease affecting the current situation. This process does not just mean that the individual needs to take extra time to recover, but that they need to do all that they can to maximise their body's healing potential, to stimulate what Hippocrates called *Vis medicatrix naturae* – the healing power of nature.

The aim of this book is to try to show natural supportive strategies and treatments that one can use in order to make the recovery pattern as near to that shown in Figure 8 as possible. You will see that this shows the ideal recovery curve with a series of spheres superimposed. Each of these spheres represents an area where a particular strategy will help. This is also the sequence in which I feel

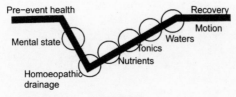

FIGURE 8

the strategies should be applied in order to aid natural recovery.

So now, please follow the chapters in their order to see how they can help one to *get well soon*.

CHAPTER 3

DON'T LET IT GET YOU DOWN

....think only of the outlook on life of the one in distress.
Dr Edward Bach

The mind and the body are inextricably linked. A negative mental state will eventually affect physical function, just as a persisting physical problem will induce a negative mental state or attitude. During recovery from an illness or health event one's mental state is crucial. Literally, *bad vibes will delay healing!* The Bach Flower Remedies are medicines which are prepared from flowers to treat the negative emotional and mental states which are common in life. In my opinion they should be an integral part of any recovery program.

DR EDWARD BACH
Dr Edward Bach was a successful homoeopath and bacteriologist attached to the Royal London Homoeopathic Hospital in the 1930s. As a research scientist he made several valuable contributions to the homoeopathic materia medica. It was therefore a huge surprise to his colleagues when he gave up both his hospital appointment and his lucrative Harley Street practice in order to begin a search for the most simple and beneficial medicines amid the woods, fields and hedgerows of the English countryside.

It was Bach's contention that people fell ill, or failed to recover from illness, because of their negative mental states. Using his research skills and his own highly developed intuition he recorded 38 negative mental states, for each of which he discovered an antidote made from the flower of a wild plant or tree.

Dr Bach divided the remedies into 7 groups:
FOR FEAR – *Rock Rose, Mimulus, Cherry Plum, Aspen, Red Chestnut.*

FOR UNCERTAINTY – *Cerato, Scleranthus, Gentian, Gorse, Hornbeam, Wild Oat.*
FOR INSUFFICIENT INTEREST IN PRESENT CIRCUMSTANCES – *Clematis, Honeysuckle, Wild Rose, Olive, White Chestnut, Mustard, Chestnut Bud.*
FOR LONELINESS – *Water Violet, Impatiens, Heather.*
FOR OVER-SENSITIVENESS – *Agrimony, Centaury, Walnut, Holly.*
FOR DESPONDENCY – *Larch, Pine, Elm, Sweet Chestnut, Star of Bethlehem, Willow, Oak, Crab Apple.*
FOR OVER-CARE FOR WELFARE OF OTHERS – *Chicory, Vervain, Vine, Beech, Rock Water.*

THE BACH FLOWER REMEDIES AND CONVALESCENCE

At the beginning of this chapter I deliberately made a pun about bad vibes affecting healing. If you think about it, this very much fits into the vibrational model I proposed in Chapter 2. Indeed, I would say that the emotional state is of fundamental importance in helping the individual to recover.

My own approach is always to assess the individual's emotional state, their mood, and their preoccupations. I look for any evidence of such emotions as guilt, anger, fear, jealousy, as well as any indication about the type of person they are. For example, I try to ascertain whether they have a rigid way of thinking, a lack of confidence, or whether they are dreamers or out and out pessimists. All of these negative states have a remedy which will remove the bad vibrations and permit healing at the higher level to begin.

Let us look at a few examples of the way the remedies can work.

CHILDBIRTH – after having a baby most women find that their emotions are in a state of flux for a time. One emotion may follow another quite inexplicably.

Feeling overwhelmed with the responsibility of becoming a mother would indicate *Elm.* Feeling extremely anxious about the baby's health when all is going well would indicate *Red Chestnut.* And having to ask everyone for their opinion, due to complete uncertainty would indicate *Cerato.*

SEVERE ILLNESS – upon having the illness diagnosed, *Star of Bethlehem* may help the acute shock. A sense of disgust about the disease process or about one's body is often helped by *Crab Apple.* Feeling introspective and sorry for oneself indicates *Willow.* Being unable to free your mind from a particular thought would indicate *White Chestnut.*

BEREAVEMENT – this can affect one profoundly, often drastically impairing one's ability to recover from an illness. A whole series of emotions occur, including shock (*Star of Bethlehem*), feeling of isolation (possibly *Impatiens*), anger (*Holly*), depression (*Mustard*) and guilt (*Pine*).

POST-OPERATIVE surgery has a profound effect on many people, partly through the physiological trauma and partly through the realisation that their body has been cut. Getting used to the idea often indicates *Walnut.* Planning the rest of one's life may lead to dilemmas, which may be helped by *Scleranthus* and *Wild Oat.*

THE INDIVIDUAL INDICATIONS

Let us now consider the full 38 indications. One needs to be quite honest about oneself in analysing the dominant negative thoughts and emotions that go through one's mind.

Agrimony – for those who hide their inner torment and feelings behind a brave face.

Aspen – for the feeling of impending doom. The fear is not something the individual can put their finger on.

Beech – for arrogant, critical people who always find fault in others. May be seething under the surface.

Centaury – the human doormat. When unable to ever say no.

Cerato – when one's own judgement cannot be depended upon. Always asking others for their opinion or judgement.

Cherry plum – for the fear that one may go insane, collapse or do something rash. This includes the impulsive suicidal type of person. They live in fear of losing control.

Chestnut Bud – for those who keep making the same mistakes in life without learning their lesson.

Chicory – for over-possessiveness. For the martyr, because they want to over-protect and care, but end up stifling the ones they care for. As a result they may be rejected and feel slighted.

Clematis – for creative, dreamy types who live in daydreams, seem indifferent and absent-minded.

Crab Apple – for self-disgust, or shame about an illness, condition, or state. It is known as the cleansing remedy.

Elm – for those who feel overwhelmed by responsibilities. A good remedy for a temporary feeling of inadequacy.

Gentian – for disappointment and discouragement. Upon hearing bad news may slump into a depression, think 'oh what's the use'.

Gorse – absolute defeatism and pessimism. This is an extreme form of Gentian. They don't bother with things because they do not believe another attempt is worth it.

Heather – talkative, chatterboxes, only interested in themselves, selfish. People may shun them and they may become lonely because they are so selfish, boring, etc.

Holly – for jealousy, anger, hatred, revenge, all the extreme negative destructive emotions. Can be explosively angry.

Honeysuckle – those who continually look back at the past, feel homesick. They live in the past with their memories.

Hornbeam – for that Monday Morning feeling. For the exhausting negative mental feeling that comes with the prospect of a difficult day or task ahead.

Impatiens – for irritability and impatience. Fidgets, always in a hurry and wants things doing yesterday.

Larch – for those lacking confidence in themselves. They expect to fail. This is different from the fear of failure or fear of loss of control of Cherry Plum.

23

Mimulus – for fear of illness, poverty, travelling, etc. It is fear of a specific thing.

Mustard – for that black depression that comes on suddenly, like a curtain being pulled down.

Oak – for those who struggle on, plod on, under any circumstance. They will often plod on when their mind and body need a rest. They never admit to feeling ill. When unable to cope they get irritable and angry with themselves!

Olive – for exhaustion, when they have used up all their energy. This is not the same as Hornbeam which may be exhausted in anticipation of the task. Olive is exhausted having done the work.

Pine – for guilt. They carry the guilt around with them, but may never be able to unburden it to anyone else.

Red Chestnut – for fear of something happening to a loved one. Not to be confused with Chicory.

Rock Rose – for terror, panic, extreme fear. Very good for nightmares and night terrors and fears following accidents or traumas.

Rock Water – for those who are strict with themselves. There is an expectation of perfection and maintenance of high (sometimes impossible) standards. Self-denying.

Scleranthus – for fluctuating moods, vacillation, indecisiveness. Always think of it in a mood swing person, the Jekyll and Hyde, the Jack and Jill, etc.

Star of Bethlehem – for acute shock or distress. After witnessing an accident, hearing bad news and so on.

Sweet Chestnut – for utter despair and anguish. When there doesn't seem to be any light at the end of the tunnel.

Vervain – for fanaticism, the outraged sense of justice. They are the missionaries, those who have to convert people to their views, principles, etc. This is different from Rock Water. Vervain may be strict, but it is to do with equality, rather than a personal strictness, as with Rock water. Will take up causes.

Vine – for domineering, inflexible, highly ambitious types.

Walnut – the link-breaker. Very useful when someone

24

needs a help in breaking a link with a place, a relationship, etc. It helps to readjust to the new situation.

Water Violet – for proud, reserved people who often seem aloof. They prefer their own company and just get on with their own lives.

White Chestnut – for those thoughts that will not go away. The mind buzz, the stuck gramophone needle in the mind. Insomnia.

Wild Oat – for the uncertainty about what to do with one's life.

Wild Rose – the drifting mentality. Prepared just to stay where one is. No ambition, no go, apathy.

Willow – for feeling sorry for oneself. Bitter and resentful, as if things always happen to me!

RESCUE REMEDY

Dr Bach advocated the use of a composite treatment (which is available over the counter) which he called the Rescue Remedy. This consists of the following:–
Cherry Plum, Clematis, Impatiens, Rock Rose and *Star of Bethlehem*. It is used in emergencies for shock, trauma, bad news, etc. and is something which should be in everyone's medicine cabinet. It is taken four drops at a time. It can also be used as a single ingredient in a treatment bottle.

USING THE BACH FLOWER REMEDIES

Once you have decided upon which remedies are indicated, you should obtain small stock bottles of these remedies from your local health shop.

To take the remedies one can take two drops directly in a small glass of water, fruit juice or even weak tea and sip it slowly. Three glasses or cups a day should soon start to lessen the negative mental state. Quite simply, you will find that the mood starts to rise and the bad feelings disappear.

It is also a good idea to make a treatment bottle up when you anticipate using it for a week or so. This is especially the case if more than one remedy is being used at a time. Indeed, you can use up to six at a time, but more than that will tend to have a lesser effect. If many emotions seem in need of treatment and alleviation, then choose the most dominant three or four and be prepared to alter the treatment bottle composition as you go along.

For your treatment bottle you need a 20 or 30 ml bottle with a dropper (available from chemists or homoeopathic suppliers). Add two drops of the remedy to the bottle then fill up with mineral water. You can add a small teaspoon of brandy if the bottle is to last for a long time. The dose is then two drops from the treatment bottle in water, fruit juice or even a cup of tea, three times a day.

I end this chapter by stating that these remedies alone may be sufficient to begin a good and full recovery process. If you get to know them well, you will never want to be without the ones that are indicated for you.

CHAPTER 4

HOMOEOPATHIC CONVALESCENT REMEDIES

*MOUNTAIN ARNICA – should be in every house, and
everybody should know of its uses.*
Dr M.L.Tyler, *Homoeopathic Drug Pictures*

Homoeopathy is a system of Medicine which is entirely stimulant, as opposed to the suppressant nature of much allopathic or Western Orthodox Medicine. Essentially, in Homoeopathy one looks at the individual's experience of their illness or condition, particularly looking at the way it makes them feel, in order to prescribe a remedy which will stimulate the innate healing ability of their own body.

Only infinitesimal amounts of the original substance are used, be that of animal, herbal or mineral origin. The remedy is usually taken in tablet form, generally for a short period of time. The theory is that once the healing power of the body has been stimulated, no more treatment is needed until the symptom pattern changes. You can think of this as being analogous to push starting a car with a flat battery. The pushing action is necessary to get the engine to fire. However, once the engine has started, the battery will charge up automatically, so that any further pushing is a waste of time.

Some homoeopathic purists believe that a single remedy should be taken at the start of an illness in order to deal with the whole illness and the recovery time. While I would not dispute that being the case when the *exact* remedy is taken, I would suggest that very often the exact indicated remedy is not the one that is prescribed. If that is the case, then a homoeopathic convalescent remedy can clear the way.

Yet I would go further than that. It is my experience

that a homoeopathic remedy can help to clear away toxins that accumulate after illness, trauma or surgery. Indeed, homoeopathic convalescent remedies form one of the simplest uses of homoeopathy.

HOMOEOPATHIC CONVALESCENT REMEDIES

In convalescence from a health event toxins of one form or another will tend to accumulate. For example, there may be cellular debris, pus formation and fluid accumulation. The main organ and organ system involved in the health event process will be most likely to accumulate these toxins. In addition, at the vibrational level, this is the part of the body's energetic field that will tend to have most disruption.

The homoeopathic convalescent remedy will help to balance the vibrational disruption to ease the energetic part of the problem. Then as a secondary effect at the tissue level the organ and organ system will start to eliminate their toxins. This will often be seen as a sort of healing crisis whereby the individual develops signs of a respiratory infection with runny nose and productive cough. In other cases there may be an increase in urine production as the urinary system is stimulated. Or then again there may be an increase in frequency of looser than usual bowel motions.

It is useful to think of these remedies having a *draining effect* during convalescence. By *draining away the toxins* that inevitably accumulate during recovery they hasten recovery.

HOW TO USE THE HOMOEOPATHIC CONVALESCENT REMEDY

Certain remedies are particularly associated with types of event and with particular organs and organ systems. One looks for the remedy associated with the type of problem or the main organ affected in the illness. The remedy should be chosen according to which keynote features most closely fit the picture.

In homoeopathy we use a number of different

potency scales. In the context of their use as convalescent remedies it is most appropriate to use the low potencies. The 6C potency (which is readily available from most health stores and many chemists) is perfectly adequate. You should obtain a small container of the remedy and take it as follows:

• The tablets should not be handled, but should be flicked into the mouth from the lid of the container, or placed there with a spoon. This is because the effectiveness of the tablet is only on the surface, not mixed all the way through as in a conventional tablet.

• Two tablets should be taken at a time, but they must be sucked not swallowed. They should be taken THREE TIMES A DAY FOR THREE DAYS ONLY.

• The tablets should not be taken within half an hour of tea, food, coffee, smoking or having brushed the teeth.

• The remedies will last for a long time, providing they are kept away from potent smelling substances. They are best kept in a drawer, away from perfumes, spices, pot-pourri or mothballs.

THE REMEDIES

The following situations and mainly affected organ are associated with the following homoeopathic convalescent remedies:

PHYSICAL TRAUMA

By this I include accidents, injuries and the trauma of surgery itself.

Aconite – when there has been agitation, excitement, restlessness and shock. The individual may have a severe persistent headache. Any exposure problem.

Arnica – where there has been much tissue damage (bruising), but generally without breakage of the skin. Excellent after broken bones and head injuries with concussion. Also of use after surgery when the individual makes light of the operation and denies that there is anything wrong.

Cantharis – extremely useful after burns to the skin.

Staphysagria – where there is anger and oversensitivity. Useful after any cutting injury. Useful after surgery where the individual is angry, aggressive and irritable.

Stramonium – useful after operations on the eye.

Symphytum – where there has been trauma causing broken bones and breakage of the skin (compound fractures).

EMOTIONAL SHOCKS AND TRAUMAS

This is a huge area, but if one aspect of the health event has been an acute emotional trauma, or if the individual is drifting into one of the adverse recovery patterns outlined in Chapter 2 then one of these four remedies may prove very effective:

Aurum – where the individual is profoundly depressed and talks of self-harm and suicide.

Causticum – where the individual is irritable, yet still manages to feel sympathetic and concerned about other people.

Ignatia – when the individual loses their cool and becomes agitated and hysterical.

Pulsatilla – when the individual is very shy, weepy and subject to changeable symptoms.

AFTER CHILDBIRTH

In days gone by women were expected to lie in, to convalesce so that the body changes of pregnancy could reverse without complication. It is now accepted that actual lying in bed for a prolonged time would put many women at risk of developing a deep vein thrombosis (DVT) which could be extremely serious. Having said that, the profound physiological changes of pregnancy can sometimes be associated with an abnormal recovery process.

Calc carb – where everything is too much of an effort and the individual feels congested in every way. They may have too much milk, be constipated and have fluid retention.

Helonias – where there are symptoms referred to the pelvis. The womb may be slow to involute or there may be a bleeding problem or persistent or recurrent infection.

Sepia – where the predominant attitude is indifference to those around them, even their baby.

THE MAIN ORGAN AFFECTED

When the main organ is easily pinpointed. Thus the lungs in a respiratory problem; the heart in a heart or cardiovascular illness and so on.

■ HEART

> *Arsenicum album* – when there is restlessness and grave anxiety
> *Baryta carb* – when there is general tiredness, a feeling of great age and a poor memory
> *Carbo veg* – where there has been collapse and faintness and severe illness
> *Crataegus* – where there is irritability, crossness and profound depression
> *Spigelia* – when there are palpitations waking one from sleep

■ LUNGS

> *Bryonia* – where there is dryness, a cough better for lying still and worse for moving
> *Carbo veg* – where there has been collapse and faintness and severe illness
> *Spongia* – where there has been much wheezing and tightness

■ NERVOUS SYSTEM

> *Gelsemium* – where there has been a general lethargy, numbness, fear and prostration
> *Ignatia* – where a hysterical reaction with hysterical fear set in

■ DIGESTIVE SYSTEM

> *Nux vomica* – for stomach problems
> *Chelidonium* – for liver and gall bladder problems
> *Ruta* – for bowels and rectum

■ **URINARY SYSTEM**

Berberis – for kidney and bladder
Thuja – for bladder and prostate

■ **SKIN**

Sulphur – for fidgety, thoughtful types with 'dirty-looking complexions'
Petroleum – for poor peripheral circulation, cracked skin and chilblain tendency

CHAPTER 5

FOOD AS MEDICINE

Let food be your medicine and medicine be your food.
Hippocrates

*A spoonful of beef-tea, or arrowroot and wine, or egg-flip
every hour will give them the required nourishment, and
prevent them from being too exhausted at a later hour to
take the solid food which is necessary.*
Florence Nightingale

The above advice given by Florence Nightingale formed the bedrock of convalescence care for many many years. Indeed, I well remember being given beef-tea according to an old family recipe when as a youthful medical student I was recuperating from a bout of glandular fever.

It is a sad fact, however, that modern Medicine has paid relatively scant attention to the role of nutrition in the recovery state. It is really fundamental that one should take food which does not tax the systems, yet which stimulates the body's healing mechanisms.

Most health events upset the body's self-regulating or homoeostatic mechanisms. Strain may be placed upon particular organs with consequent build-up of metabolic end-products. The body's attempts to heal itself involves the use of compensatory mechanisms which remove the strain from the straining organ or system, and the removal of the build-up of toxins.

In the recovery phase after a health event the role of nutrition is to give the body the essential foods which aid the recovery process, but without giving it foodstuffs which can hamper that process. In particular it is important not to take in foods which throw an added strain upon the system or which impede the elimination of the toxic end-products of metabolism.

THE ESSENTIAL FOODS

The essentials of any diet are water, protein, fat, carbohydrate and fibre, minerals and vitamins.

PROTEIN is an essential part of the diet, since every enzyme in the body is a protein structure. That being the case, there is not a chemical reaction within the living cell which is not dependent upon proteins.

In addition to making enzymes, proteins are involved in blood clotting mechanisms. The antibodies that fight infections and maintain immunity in the body are proteins. Fat and cholesterol is transported around the body by proteins. And also, significantly, proteins form the structure of muscles, tendons, arteries and veins.

One great problem for the body, however, is the fact that it cannot synthesise all the proteins needed from the basic building bricks called *amino acids*. There are 22 basic amino acids, but the body can only make some of them. The rest have to be furnished from the diet. The ones which the body can make are called *non-essential amino acids*. The remaining eight, which must be absorbed from the diet, are called *essential amino-acids*.

Foods that contain all eight essential amino acids in the proportions needed by the body are called high-quality proteins. These are usually derived from:

animal or dairy products. Plant foods usually do not contain as much high-quality protein, exceptions being *soya beans, tofu, corn, peas, peanuts, Brewer's yeast and wheat germ.*

FATS are a group of large, insoluble molecules which have a very high energy content. Unlike proteins which are made up of repeated amino acids, fats are made up of glycerol, fatty acids, triglycerides and cholesterol. The fatty acids are the important parts, because they are needed in the production of cell membranes, certain hormones and the sheaths which surround nerves.

Like proteins, however, the body cannot manufacture all of the fatty acids. Two types – the *linoleic acid* and *alpha-linoleic acid* groups – are called *essential fatty acids*. They have to be obtained from the diet.

The ideal source of these fatty acids can be found in the following oils: *safflower-seed oil, evening primrose oil, olive oil, sunflower oil, soya bean oil or corn oil.*

CARBOHYDRATE is the name given to a group of organic compounds which include starch, polysaccharides and simple sugars.

While the body must have proteins and some fat for fatty acids, it does not, in recovery, need much in the way of carbohydrates. They do not regulate metabolic processes as do proteins. Indeed, their main function in a diet is to produce energy for the metabolic processes.

In convalescence carbohydrates are best taken in the form of *complex carbohydrates*. These are carbohydrates containing both starch and dietary fibre. The latter consists of the supporting tissue of plants. It is of great benefit to the functioning of the bowel, as well as having a role in keeping cholesterol and blood glucose levels down.

Such foods are *wholegrain cereals, pulses, fruit and vegetables.*

A raw source of simple sugars, such as honey, is preferable to loading the system with refined sugars. (see Chapter 6).

FIBRE As mentioned above, fibre is important for helping the bowel to function. It consists of complex sugars which are not significantly digested by the body. It is supplied totally from plants, so it is vital that it is included within the diet in convalescence.

In health, the normal intake of fibre in the UK is only 12 grams per day. This is woefully inadequate and should be nearer 30 grams. One should be aiming at increasing to this figure in convalescence.

Fibre is best taken naturally, rather than in the form of laxatives and fibre supplements. That way the bowel will be able to develop a natural way of dealing with it. However, care must be taken in gradually increasing the fibre content of the diet, since it will provoke gas retention and abdominal bloating if there is a sudden change in dietary intake. In addition, one must ensure a good fluid intake at the same time, because the fibre passing undigested through the bowel will take more fluid with it.

MINERALS are important in all aspects of metabolism.
Calcium and Phosphorus – bone metabolism. Found in: *milk, cheese, yoghurt, oily fish and flour.*
Magnesium – protein synthesis. Found in *wholegrains, green vegetables, nuts.*
Iron – blood production. Found in *red meat, liver, shellfish, lentils, wholemeal bread.*
Sodium – fluid balance and functioning of kidney, nerves and muscles. Found in *bread, salted foods.* Take care not to add in convalescence.
Potassium – fluid balance and heart, kidney, muscle and nerve functioning. Found in *green vegetables, mushrooms, potatoes, tomatoes, grapes, Brewer's yeast.*
Chloride – fluid and acid-base balance. Found with sodium in *salt.*
Fluoride – this is an important trace element, mainly found in teeth and bones. Found in *tea and seaweeds.*
Iodine – this is an essential trace mineral necessary for thyroid gland function. Found in *seaweed, dairy products, fish.*
Selenium – this is an essential trace element which complements Vitamin E as an antioxidant (see below). It is found in *fish, cheese, eggs, nuts and wholemeal bread.*
Zinc – this important trace element is needed to help in countless enzymatic reactions within the body. It is also important in fertility in both sexes, and in wound healing. Found in *nuts, vegetables, wholegrains and pulses.*

VITAMINS are organic substances needed by the body in minute amounts for a whole host of bodily processes. The term comes from the latin *vita*, meaning life and *amine*, the name for a type of chemical.

There are about 20 vitamins which have to be taken in the diet, because the body cannot synthesise them. Most vitamins are destroyed by cooking, so fresh, raw or par-cooked foods yield the greatest amounts.

Some vitamins are fat soluble. These can actually prove troublesome if too much is taken into the system, when they can be toxic. Vitamins A, D, E and K are fat soluble. The body cannot easily get rid of them so they are retained in fat stores.

Vitamins C and the B group are water soluble, so do not cause this problem.

Vitamin A – needed for growth, night sight, cell membranes. Available in *animal foods, particularly liver, in active form of retinol. Available in plants as a precursor, beta-carotene.*

Vitamin B group – these are necessary for all sorts of metabolic functioning. Also important for nerve development. Folic Acid is necessary for pregnant women to prevent neural tube defects (spina bifida, etc.) Available in *meats, cheese, liver, fish, wholegrains, vegetables, bananas, avocados and Brewer's yeast,* or as a *Vitamin B compound tablet.*

Vitamin C – ascorbic acid, available in *all citrus fruits and fresh vegetables.* Needed to help build blood and maintain integrity of connective tissue.

Vitamin D – the sunshine vitamin, which is manufactured in the body. Also available in *oily fish.* It is necessary for calcium metabolism.

Vitamin E – an important antioxidant, which is necessary for maintaining cell membranes. Extremely beneficial to the circulation. Available in *wheat germ oil, vegetable oils, leafy vegetables and poly-unsaturated margarines.*

Vitamin K – an essential vitamin for helping the co-agulation system of the blood. There are three types of Vitamin K – Vitamin K_1, K_2 and K_3. Vitamin K_1 is present in *oils like soya, green vegetables and liver.* The other two can be manufactured by the body.

ANTIOXIDANTS

One of the most interesting theories of modern Medicine concerns the problems caused by *free radicals.* Basically, free radicals are molecules with unpaired electrons. They occur during all sorts of metabolic processes in the body, and have the capability of damaging DNA, enzymes, proteins and fats, through the process of oxidation. The problem then is that cell membranes and delicate cell organelles can be damaged or destroyed resulting in tissue impairment.

After a health event there is likely to be an increase in free radicals with the potential of producing even further damage during recovery. If nothing else, the tissue impairment will be likely to result in an accumulation of toxins.

The process of oxidation is rather like the fatigue and rotting that occurs in an elastic band left exposed to the atmosphere. If you imagine this taking place in delicate blood vessels and tissues then you can see how dangerous it can become.

Fortunately, the effect of free radicals can be minimised and to some degree nullified by naturally occurring antioxidants. These are substances such as Vitamin E, carotene (the name for a group of substances which can be converted in the body into Vitamin A), various enzymes and Vitamin C. The main sources of these are *nuts, fruit and vegetables*, especially raw ones. Particularly rich are many of the foods with a bright orange or red colour, such as *carrots, apricots, pumpkin, cantaloupe melon, and red peppers.* All of these should be eaten freely.

The value of nuts has been demonstrated in research from America. A handful of nuts (*peanuts, almonds or walnuts*) five times a week reduces the risk of having a heart attack by half. They are extremely valuable after a health event, particularly one caused by a degenerative disease.

FOOD IN CONVALESCENCE

In the UK in the 1990s 42% of the energy in the average adult diet comes from fat, 41% from carbohydrate, 11% from protein and 6% from alcohol. This is far from ideal and for most people it is advisable that fat should contribute less that 35%. Carbohydrate should be boosted to 50%, while protein should remain the same at 11%. Alcohol should be restricted to 5%.

After a health event when the appetite may have been lost and the absorptive ability of the body has been impaired, it is important to modify this even further. One should not overload the body with too much fat. Cutting the level to 25–30% of the dietary energy intake is desirable as is increasing protein to 15–20%. The carbohydrate intake is best taken in the form of complex carbohydrates which contain starch and fibre. These are to be found in wholegrains, pulses, vegetables and fruits.

Rather than giving examples of an ideal recovery diet (which there isn't), one should consider the principles of a good diet. To assist, you should look at the following DO's and DON'Ts

DO

• Take proteins from white meat, fish, free-range eggs, lentils, soya, yoghurt (preferably live yoghurt), cheese, nuts, beans and tofu. In particular try to take oily fish (salmon, trout, mackerel, sardines or herring) three times a week.

• Use complex carbohydrates from unrefined wholemeal cereals, porridge oats, wholemeal bread, potatoes, pulses and vegetables.

• Use raw vegetables in salads. Cooking destroys

many vitamins and causes leaching out of important minerals. Par-boil vegetables for cooked meals and use the strained juice for making gravies or as a drink in itself.

• Ensure a daily intake of antioxidant containing vegetables. Remember the orange or red 'marker'.

• Take fresh fruit every day. At least two pieces should be eaten daily.

• Take a handful of dried fruit three times a week.

• Take a handful of nuts (walnuts, unsalted peanuts, almonds) three times a week.

• Use extra virgin olive oil for cooking, adding to salads or for soaking baked potatoes in. Alternatively, use sunflower oil or corn oil.

• Use good quality mineral water rather than tap water.

• Use fresh milk, fresh fruit juice and freshly squeezed vegetable juice (if a juicer is available) daily.

DON'T

• Don't Smoke. Many people find that a health event provides them with the opportunity and the impetus to stop. Do try stopping, since the toxicity of tobacco smoking will certainly impede the body's natural healing, since it increases the amount of free radicals.

• Don't drink too much alcohol. Keep intake to the bare minimum. Try to regard it as a treat not a necessity. Allow a glass of alcohol up to three times a week. Preferably this should be in the form of wine rather than beer or spirits.

• Don't eat red meat. Preferably avoid it altogether. If you need to take meat then make sure that it is white and lean (unless using it as a source of an essential mineral or vitamin).

• Don't eat refined and processed foods.

• Don't eat chocolate and confectionary.

• Don't take chemical food flavourings and colourings. These tend to add to the pool of toxins that are liable to accumulate during convalescence. Avoid fizzy, coloured soft drinks.

• Don't eat tinned, smoked and pickled foods.
• Do not add salt or sugar to foods or drinks. If sweetening is needed use a raw sugar form, like honey.

SPECIAL FOODS IN DIFFERENT TYPES OF CONVALESCENCE

So far you will note that the only supplement to the diet which I would recommend in convalescence is Vitamin B compound. I think that the dietary principles outlined above are more important. Observe these and you will find that you take in adequate amounts of nutrients, minerals and vitamins. However, in the convalescence from particular types of health event, certain additional foods or drinks will help.

In the following groups of illnesses, the foods that are especially indicated should be taken three times a week at least and preferably daily.

INFECTIONS AND INFECTIOUS ILLNESSES

The immune system will have been affected and needs help to build its reserves again. This is particularly the case if there has been much dosing with antibiotics. The following are beneficial:

Yoghurt, garlic, onions, mushrooms, carrots, red peppers, walnuts, shellfish.

HEART AND CIRCULATORY PROBLEMS

Here it is important to avoid further damage from fats, smoking and excess alcohol. The following are beneficial:

Fresh fruit, dried raisins, prunes, red vegetables including carrots, red peppers, walnuts, olive oil, garlic and onions.

RESPIRATORY PROBLEMS

Severe asthma, emphysema, and other conditions producing breathlessness of respiratory origin are often eased by the following foods:

Garlic, onions, hot peppers and spices, fresh fruit, fish.

STOMACH PROBLEMS

Upper gastro-intestinal problems, including heartburn and ulceration of the stomach and duodenum may be aided by the following:

Bananas, cabbage, liquorice, raw potatoes.

GALL BLADDER PROBLEMS

Here the avoidance of fat in animal meat and dairy products is important. The following are beneficial:

Fresh vegetables, fresh oranges, soya, olive oil.

LARGE BOWEL PROBLEMS

Irritable bowel syndrome, diverticular disease, colitis and other inflammatory problems may be helped by:

Bran, wholefood cereals, fresh fruit and live yoghurt.

KIDNEY AND URINARY PROBLEMS

One should avoid refined foods. The following are beneficial:

Fresh fruits, cranberry juice, brown rice, broccoli, figs, shellfish.

GYNAECOLOGICAL PROBLEMS

Taking phyto-oestrogens in the diet may be particularly helpful for people troubled with many gynaecological problems including PMS, painful periods, and menopausal symptoms. The most convenient form is by taking Linseed oil capsules (2–5 per day), or one of the sprouting legumes or beansprouts.

The following are also often beneficial:

Bananas, apricots, lentils, beans, oats, oil of evening primrose.

POST SURGERY

This is often helped by the foods under the appropriate headings given above. The following are also often beneficial:

Fresh citrus fruits, kelp tablets, orange-red vegetables including red peppers, carrots and cantaloupe melon, walnuts.

ARTHRITIC PROBLEMS

The following are often beneficial:

Oily fish, fresh leafy vegetables, ginger root.

EMOTIONAL PROBLEMS

Depression can be aided by:

Spinach, seafood, garlic.

Anxiety states may be aided by:

Wholefoods, raw sugars like honey.

NOTE: *IF ONE SUSPECTS A FOOD ALLERGY OR SENSITIVITY, THEN ADVICE FROM A DOCTOR OR NUTRITIONIST SHOULD BE OBTAINED FIRST.*

CHAPTER 6

NATURAL TONICS

*'The power of herbs and their value for curing
purposes....'*
Virgil, *Aeneid*

Tonics have been prepared by people since Medicine began. Essentially, they are remedies which are thought to 'tone up' the system. They can be extremely valuable when trying to hasten recovery from an illness, to boost the immune system, or to just give that bit more energy.

Most of the tonics which follow are readily available either in one's kitchen cupboard or from a health food shop or herbal supplier. You will find that they are supplied loose or as 'tea bags'. Thus, they are easily taken as herbal teas or tisanes, or as additives to a tisane. They can be taken once or twice a day for the first week or two, then gradually spacing out as recovery is achieved. Ideally, if one can get used to them, they are much better for you than drinking coffee.

GENERAL TONICS

This group of tonics have a general toning up effect. They are of value after a debilitating infection, childbirth, operation or accident.

HONEY – I start with this food, because it ranks top of my personal list of tonics. Not only that, its pedigree is as long as you can get. There is a legend that when Hippocrates died they placed a beehive on his tomb, because he had extolled the value of honey for many years. The honey which the bees produced from that hive was thought to be especially effective.

While diabetics should avoid all sugars and have their diets guided by their doctors, for mostly everyone else honey is an excellent food. In the convalescent stages of illness or after an operation, I think that a dessertspoonful of honey twice a day can work wonders. It is also an idea to take it in a herbal infusion or tisane, since it will help to ease the bitterness of many such drinks.

It can also be taken as 'Hydromel', which is basically a mixture of honey, water, and various spices. The choice of spice is up to the individual's taste, but I rather like cinnamon. Mead is of course a fermented variety of hydromel. A small glass a day is a good pick-me-up after a debilitating illness.

GINSENG – This herb (*Panax ginseng*) also has a long pedigree as a tonic. The botanical name Panax is derived from the Greek *Panakes*, meaning 'all-healing' – (similar to our word panacea). This is a warming herb which really does lift one's energy. It is extremely bitter and may benefit from the addition of a spoonful of honey or some chopped liquorice root. A cup morning and evening is the recommended dosage.

KELP – This tonic agent has a remarkable reputation. It is a seaweed (*Fucus vesiculosis*), also called Bladderwrack, which has been used as a laxative, a tonic, a slimming agent and a thyroid gland stabiliser. It is rich in Iodine.

I have found this to be an effective aid in rheumatic disorders and a good all round tonic. It is readily available in health shops in tablet form. It is not one for prolonged self-treatment, however. It should be taken under the advice of a health professional.

Up to three tablets a day can be taken, in the dosage of 5–10 grams of the dried herb equivalent.

BASIL – (*Ocimum basilicum*) This is an excellent restorative when one is exhausted. A sprig of basil leaves infused in a pint of water makes an excellent tisane.

CALCIUM TINCTURE – This tonic is traditionally taken to aid the healing of bones. In these days of the 'modern epidemic' of osteoporosis, it may also help with calcium balance.

Take the shells of a dozen eggs, dry them and remove the inner membranes so that you simply have the calcium shells. Pulverise and powder them and add to 600 ml or a pint of cider vinegar. There will be a lot of froth created so use a large container. Add 50 grams of honey and mix well. Keep the tincture in a screw-cap container, plastic preferably, in case of excessive pressure, and keep releasing the pressure until the tincture is flat.

Two tablespoonfuls three times a day is the recommended dosage after food. This should be taken with care, however, by anyone who suffers from dyspepsia or stomach ulceration.

CARROT JUICE – (*Daucus carota*) Although carrots are not easy to juice, the effort is well worthwhile. A glass of this tonic juice as and when one needs a pick-me-up works well indeed.

CAYENNE – (*Capsicum minimum*) When a bit of extra zest or 'pep' is needed, try adding a pinch of cayenne pepper to a herbal tisane.

PEPPERMINT – (*Mentha piperita*), is a well-known general tonic. An infusion as a herbal tea is good for relieving congested headaches, stimulating the stomach and easing the pain of varicose veins.

CIRCULATORY TONICS

These tonics are worth taking in convalescence after a circulatory problem, or if hypertension is a problem. GARLIC – (*Allium sativum*) This herb was known to the Ancient Egyptians, Chinese, Greeks and Romans. Garlic cloves have apparently been found in Ancient Egyptian tombs, left there as tonics to restore the Ka of the departed in the afterlife.

Garlic is a natural antibiotic and is of value in hypertension and circulatory problems. It is excellent for the digestive system and is a good tonic in convalescent states. It can be taken several ways. It can be cooked in food, chewed as the clove, or swallowed as garlic capsules. Parsley is worth chewing afterwards in order to counter the characteristic pungent garlic odour.

CAYENNE PEPPER – (*Capsicum annum*) is used as a tonic for the heart, for aching legs and sluggish circulation. About a quarter of a teaspoon is taken in a cup of hot water twice a day for as long as felt necessary. This is best taken after food. Once improvement occurs, the treatment is stopped.

ROSE – (*Rosacea*) is an ancient remedy for the heart. Traditionally, two dessertspoonfuls of the rose petals should be crushed and mixed thoroughly with one dessertspoonful of honey. This is left outside for twenty-four hours to soak up the energies of the moon and the sun. A stock should then be made (from the above quantities mixed with a pint of boiling water) and a dessertspoonful taken every morning.

RESPIRATORY TONICS

In recovery from a respiratory illness there is often a need for a remedy which will help to soothe catarrh as well as act as a tonic.

MUSTARD – (*Sinapsis alba*), also called Gold Dust, can clear catarrh and bronchitis when a weak infusion is sipped sparingly throughout the day. Too much will overheat the stomach and induce nausea. It is, however, a highly stimulating tonic.

ELECAMPANE – (*Inula helenium*), also called Wild Sunflower and Horseheal, is useful for respiratory catarrh and for clearing up bronchitis when taken as a herbal tea.

DIGESTIVE TONICS

These tonics are excellent for helping the digestive tract.

LIQUORICE – (*Glycyrrhiza glabra*) This herb contains a compound which is steroid-like, or rather like the hormone ACTH (Adrenocorticotrophic hormone), which stimulates the cortex of the adrenal gland to produce its steroidal hormones. It therefore has anti-inflammatory effects, antispasmodic and ulcer healing effects. It is quite superb for gastric problems and dyspepsia. It is also a potent laxative.

It is commonly used to flavour herbal remedies and can be taken in herbal teas to remove some of the bitterness.

The dried root can be chewed directly, or the grated

root taken in a dose of 1–4 grams of the root three times a day in a neutral solution. It can also be taken grated in other herbal infusions.

NOTE: *CARE HAS TO BE TAKEN IN PEOPLE WHO RETAIN FLUID, SINCE IT CAN ENHANCE THIS EFFECT WITH POTENTIALLY HARMFUL RESULTS. IT SHOULD NOT, THEREFORE, BE TAKEN BY PEOPLE SUFFERING FROM HEART PROBLEMS OR HYPERTENSION.*

ANISEED – (*Pimpinella anisum*) This is an excellent digestive tonic and appetite stimulant. The seeds can be chewed or taken in an infusion. Alternatively, a small glass of the liqueur once a day can be taken if preferred!

CINNAMON – (*Cinnamomum zeylanicum*) is used for stimulating the digestive system when there is thought to be sluggishness. It is taken like cayenne, as a pinch in another herbal tea or in a cup of hot water, for as long as felt necessary.

DANDELION – (*Taraxacum officinale*), also called *Devil's Milk-Pail*, is a well known bitter which has been used for digestive problems for centuries. It is effective as a laxative, diuretic and also as an aid to slimming. The leaves can be freely chewed, although over-indulgence can cause nausea. An infusion of the leaves taken as a herbal tea is also quite a useful way of taking the herb. As yet another alternative, the dried roots, ground and powdered can make a coffee substitute.

FENNEL – (*Foeniculum vulgare*) is useful for settling constipation, for enhancing fertility and for helping rheumatism. It is also reputed to be helpful in dealing with obesity. An infusion can be taken as a tisane every other day.

ARTHRITIC TONICS
When arthritic or rheumatic problems have been part of the debility, then the following two tonics are worth trying.

CIDER VINEGAR – This remedy was made famous by Dr D.C. Jarvis, in his book *Folk Medicine,* which was first published in the 1950s. Dr Jarvis practised in Vermont for some fifty years, during which time he studied Folk Medicine. He concluded that two tea-spoonfuls of Cider vinegar and two spoonfuls of honey in a glass of water at each meal works as a natural tonic. He particularly felt that it worked well in arthritic conditions.

I would certainly accept that this is an excellent tonic which is very useful in some arthritic sufferers. I would counsel care, however, if someone suffers from stomach trouble, since the vinegar, being acidic, can cause dyspepsia or a flare-up of a peptic ulcer.

NETTLE – (*Urtica urens*), the Common Stinging Nettle, also called Bad Man's Plaything, and Sting-leaf, makes a useful tisane for arthritis and rheumatic problems. An infusion taken as a herbal tea is taken once or twice a day.

GYNAECOLOGICAL TONICS

These tonics are useful after gynaecological surgery, debility from heavy painful periods, and after gynaeco-logical infections.

LINSEED OIL – This tonic is one which I have found to be very effective for easing the tiredness and flush-ing of the menopause. It is derived from Flax (*Linum usitatissimum*) and is rich in phyto-oestrogens, which are compounds which resemble female oestrogen. Research studies have shown that when linseed oil capsules are taken regularly by menopausal women, there is a significant reduction in flushing and vaginal dryness. These are actually the two only real symp-toms of the climacteric or menopause which can be said to be due to oestrogen lack. It is available in capsule form from most health shops, the dosage being one to three capsules a day.

In addition to this, it has antispasmodic effects which help to ease period pains.

RASPBERRY LEAF – (*Rubus idaeus*) The tonic effect

of Raspberry leaf tea upon the female womb is well known in the last weeks of pregnancy. It is available in tea-bag form.

YARROW – (*Achillea millefolium*), also called Blood-wort, Woundwort and Staunch-weed, is another herb which is good for easing sluggish and irregular periods, easing period pains and for stimulating the appetite. It is taken as a herbal tisane every day until recovery is noted.

URINARY TONICS

HORSE-RADISH – (*Armoracia rusticana*) is used as a remedy to stimulate the appetite, expel worms and parasites and relieve urinary tract infections. As a tonic, one or two roots can be grated down and taken once a day before the main meal. Taking bread at the same time will reduce the heat in one's mouth.

BARLEY WATER – This is an excellent household remedy for many urinary problems, since it alters the pH of the urine and soothes the urinary mucosa. It is also an appetite stimulant in the recovery from a urinary tract illness and works as a mild tonic.

Ingredients: 100 grams of pearl barley (approx 4 ounces); 50 grams of honey (approx 2 ounces); the juice from half a squeezed lemon; 600 ml of water (1 pint).

The barley is scalded then simmered in a pint of boiled water to which is added the lemon juice. Once the barley goes soft it can be removed from the heat and (after straining off the barley) the honey be added. A cup three times a day is taken for relief of the symptoms of frequency and dysuria (painful passage of urine).

As a tonic it can be taken twice a day in recovery from a urinary problem.

TONICS FOR BLOOD PROBLEMS

Anaemia is common after blood loss from accidents, surgery, childbirth and heavy periods. The exact diagnosis is important, because different conventional treatments will restore the blood to normality. In addition to plenty of citrus fruits containing vitamin C (which helps the absorption of iron), the following tonics seem to help.

AGRIMONY TEA – (*Agrimonia eupatoria*) Two heaped spoonfuls of agrimony leaves to three quarters of a pint of boiling water should be infused for half a minute, before straining. Two cups a day should be drunk.

CHICORY ROOT – (*Cichorium intybus*) is available as a coffee substitute. Two cups a day.

NETTLE – (*Urtica urens*), the Common Stinging Nettle, also called Bad Man's Plaything, and Sting-leaf, makes a useful tisane which is tonic to the blood. An infusion taken as a herbal tea is taken once or twice a day.

CHAPTER 7

WATER TO THE RESCUE

*The bath is useful in many diseases, in some of them
when used steadily, and in others when not so....*
Hippocrates

Water is the prime essential of life. No-one can do without it for any great length of time. We are essentially fluid creatures, some eighty per cent of our bodies being made up of fluid. And just as we begin life in a fluid environment, so does our every metabolic reaction depend upon water.

Many conditions affect our fluid intake and our fluid output. If you lose more than you take in you become dehydrated. If you retain more than is needed, you put on weight and parts of the body become oedematous or puffy. The actual treatment of the ailment should have restored the physiological balance. In the recovery state after the illness or health event it is up to the individual to do all that he can to ensure that the fluid balance is not compromised.

When the body is functioning properly the homoeostatic mechanisms operate so that the intake of fluid in drinks and food is matched by the output in perspiration, urine and faeces. In a country such as the UK, about two litres of fluid a day is about the required intake for a healthy adult.

DRINKS

Water is the best drink of all. Human nature being as it is, however, relatively few people are satisfied just drinking water. They prefer taking flavoured drinks, often containing stimulants of one form or another.

Water is variable, however. In the UK the water sources are generally safe from infectious agents, which still pose a significant health hazard in many countries of the world.

Different areas also produce water of varying hardness. *Hard water* contains more salts of calcium and other minerals than does soft water. This is apparent in that hard water does not lather with soap and is prone to deposit fur in kettles and water pipes. By contrast, *soft water* lathers well and produces little furring of pipes and containers. This is partly due to the fact that soft water is more acidic than hard water and tends to actually dissolve lead and other metals from pipes.

Although we are as yet unsure of the actual mechanism, it is also clinically observed that areas which have soft water tend to have higher rates of heart disease. This finding alone tends to make one wary of drinking tap water from soft water areas. Indeed, if one has had a circulatory problem, then soft water consumption may be a contributory factor. That being the case, one would be well advised, in my opinion, to obtain a water filter or to drink mineral water alone.

Natural spring water is, as the name implies, naturally occurring water obtained from some underground spring. Of course, the area it comes from will have its own properties, but the concentration of the minerals is legally limited to no more than 2 grams per litre. Most spring waters will contain calcium, magnesium, potassium and sodium as bicarbonates and sulphates. Their great advantage is in not having added chlorine or fluoride, and they will not contain dissolved lead or aluminium. They can be either carbonated or still. Whichever you choose is up to personal preference.

A water filter is a cheaper alternative and is a good addition to your kitchen. They can be attached directly to the cold drinking tap, or used in the form of a jug and filter.

In convalescence it is advisable to take half of your daily fluid intake as mineral or filtered water. Ideally the rest should be taken as fruit juice or one of the herbal teas mentioned in Chapter 6.

Coffee and tea should be restricted as much as

possible during convalescence, taking no more than two cups of either per day (two cups total, not two of each!).

Alcohol is a good vasodilator, so it can help recovery. Again, it should be used as a treat and not a regular part of recovery. I would suggest no more than a single drink every other day. Finally, wine is better than beer. Distilled alcohol on the other hand can have a deleterious effect and is best avoided during convalescence.

THE REMEDIAL EFFECTS OF BATHING

People often think that a good hot bath or a shower is an excellent way of freshening up. Indeed, during convalescence from a health event when one may have been perspiring more than usual, or just not felt like washing, there is a tendency to have too many hot baths or showers. The result is that one often feels worse, more tired and quite uncomfortable.

Baths and showers can play a very useful part in convalescence, provided you understand the underlying principles. There are in fact three ways in which water and bathing can exert a remedial effect upon the body. Through the action of temperature on the skin, by the mechanical effects of water and rubbing, and by the subtle action of the additives in medicated baths.

1) THE SKIN AND TEMPERATURE

The skin is an extremely important organ in its own right. It is ninety per cent responsible for regulating the temperature of the body. It protects the inner tissues and organs from the outer environment and manufactures Vitamin D under the action of sunlight. But in addition it also has absorption and excretory functions. For this latter reason it is often called *the third kidney.*

The circulation to and within the skin takes up ten per cent of the blood volume of the body. Under the action of the autonomic nervous system the skin blood vessels – *the arterioles, capillaries and venules* – can be dilated or constricted. This effect can be profound, since it can markedly increase or decrease the amount of blood flowing through the skin. This obviously will affect the circulation to other deeper organs and structures.

When heat in any form is applied to the skin there is a reflex dilation of the skin blood vessels. This increased blood flow becomes obvious as reddening, flushing or blushing of the skin. This is afterwards followed by increased perspiration and loss of heat from the body. Conversely, when the skin is cooled there is a reflex constriction of the skin blood vessels. This decreased flow causes pallor, inhibition of perspiration and ultimately shivering.

Whatever happens to the skin circulation automatically has an effect upon the internal organs. When external heat causes more blood to be diverted to the skin, the supply to the deeper tissues and internal organs is reduced. The autonomic circulation brings in compensatory mechanisms to deal with this. This may result in temporary reduction in function. For example, the gastro-intestinal tract activity is reduced, the pelvic organs relax and the nervous system is sedated.

In addition, moist heat, as from a bath, is extremely good for easing muscle spasm and the pain which often results from it.

When the skin is cooled, the opposite effects can be expected. The supply of blood to the deeper tissues and organs is increased.

Perspiration

The main method by which the body loses its heat is through perspiration. If the body is immersed in water or wrapped so that the perspiration cannot evaporate, then this causes the heating effect upon the skin to become even more profound. When the perspiration is finally allowed to take place, after leaving the water, the excretory function of the skin comes into action. *The third kidney* will help to remove accumulated toxins. This detoxification function of the skin can be very beneficial in convalescence.

Temperature ranges

Different temperatures have different effects upon the body. In some circumstances a hot application will help, while at other times it will make matters worse. Three temperature ranges are particularly important: *cold, tepid and hot.*

Cold – (50°–85°F; 10°–29°C) These temperatures are used to stimulate metabolism, diminish muscle irritability (after the shivering stops), tone up the skin, increase immunity. These temperatures should only be used by fit people with no heart or blood pressure problems. This is because the cold can produce an alteration in heart rate and a short rise in blood pressure.

The very lowest temperatures should only be used for a few seconds at a time. At the higher end of the range the maximum time should be two minutes.

Tepid – (85°–97°F; 29°–36°C) This range of temperature is similar to body temperature (98.4°F or 37°C), so we are not expecting profound physiological changes. There will not be much perspiration caused, so there will be little excretion of toxins, and there will not be stimulation of metabolism from the cold reaction.

The main remedial function of the tepid bath is to create a pleasant temperature for the individual to soak in water which has been medicated.

A tepid bath can be tolerated without undue problem for fifteen minutes to an hour.

Hot – (100°–107°F; 38°–41°C) This range is used when one wishes to stimulate the excretory role of the skin, to stimulate the 'third kidney' to aid detoxification.

This range is also very useful for the pain-killing effect the heat produces on muscles and joints. It is also beneficial for many problems associated with painful spasm-type pain. Finally, the hot bath has a sedating and relaxing effect. For this reason it is best taken later in the day when one can lie down afterwards. It is beneficial in tension states and when troubled by insomnia.

They can be taken for between five and fifteen minutes, but should ideally be restricted to such times that the individual does not have to leave the house after them.

2) MECHANICAL EFFECTS UPON THE BODY

Archimedes' principle states that when a body is immersed in water it displaces its own weight. Because the body is not so heavy in water, it is easier to move the limbs. Exercise in water is therefore excellent when there is restriction of movement from weakness or pain.

Water obviously washes the surface of the skin. This is useful when removing metabolic waste, but less desirable if it is reducing natural body oils. The individual should not bathe more than is necessary. In general there is no need to bathe more than once a day. This is particularly important with hot baths, since they have an enhanced excretory potential. Quite simply, too many hot baths will deplete one's vitality and predispose to debility.

Counter-irritation of the skin: It is a fact that if one has a painful condition, it is possible to stimulate fine nerve supplies in the skin in such a way that their stimulation will override the painful impulses from the main pain condition. This may be one of the mechanisms of action of various showers, jacuzzis and douches. It may also explain the mode of action of some types (though not all) of medicated bath.

3) MEDICATED BATHS

The third means by which bathing can exert a remedial effect is through the use of additives to the bath. As mentioned above, some exert a counter-irritation effect. Others work by absorption of the substance through the skin. During convalescence the most useful additives are those which exert a subtle effect upon the body's healing mechanisms – essential aromatherapy oils.

BATHING IN CONVALESCENCE

During convalescence there are two types of problem that bathing can help. Firstly, depleted energy from the illness. Secondly, diminished well-being from the build up of toxins from the illness and/or the treatment.

I am first of all going to assume that the individual is able to have and is able to get into a bath.

1) DEPLETED ENERGY

This is extremely common. One feels low in energy after many illnesses because the immune system has been burning up energy. After childbirth one's physiology is returning to normal after several months of pregnancy and the sheer work of the labour. After surgery one's body is reaccustoming itself to the surgical alteration that has been created in the body's anatomy.

One can either stimulate the energy levels by having a cold bath every morning for up to two minutes, or, probably more acceptably, by having a tepid aromatherapy bath every morning for ten to fifteen minutes.

Note that the morning is specified. This is because it is the most stimulatory part of the day.

The temperature range for a cold bath is 50°–85°F (10°–29°C), but realistically one should have it nearer the 85°F figure.

An aromatherapy bath is taken in the temperature range of 85°–97°F (29°–36°C). To this bath one adds 6–8 drops of the appropriate aromatherapy oil.

CIRCULATORY PROBLEMS – *Ylang Ylang, Lavender, Rose or Rosemary* are all effective in convalescence from heart and circulatory problems.
RESPIRATORY PROBLEMS – *Basil, Elecampane, Eucalyptus, Hyssop, Lavender and Sandalwood* are all effective in convalescence from a respiratory illness.

DIGESTIVE PROBLEMS – *Chamomile, Cypress, Lavender, Marjoram, or Peppermint* are useful in convalescence from a digestive ailment.

URINARY PROBLEMS – *Juniper, Sandalwood or Tea-tree oil* are all effective in convalescence from a urinary problem.

GYNAECOLOGICAL PROBLEMS – *Chamomile, Clary Sage, Cypress, Geranium, Jasmine, Lavender or Rose* are all effective in convalescence from a gynaeco-logical problem.

POST NATALLY – *Fennel, Geranium and Lavender* may all help restore energy after childbirth, as well as aid breastfeeding.

ARTHRITIC PROBLEMS – *Juniper, Lavender, Rosemary or Thyme* are all effective in convalescence where arthritic or rheumatic problems have been part of the health event.

EMOTIONAL PROBLEMS – *Chamomile, Jasmine, Sandalwood and Ylang Ylang* may aid anxiety states.

– *Lavender, Rose and Sandalwood* may aid depressive problems.

– *Chamomile, Lavender, Rose, Sandalwood and Ylang Ylang* are all effective for sleep problems.

2) TOXIN BUILD-UP

In this situation you are dealing with the build-up of toxins from the illness process and the body reaction. Possibly you are also dealing with the toxin build-up as a result of treatment.

One should be in no doubt about this, some treat-ments, because of the potency of the drugs used, do of their own accord produce toxin build-ups. Convalescence therefore depends upon getting over the health event and getting over the effect of the treat-ment. That is, until the drug residues and their effects are removed, the individual will feel below par.

This is a good method for dealing with the malaise from taking antibiotics, antimicrobials, chemotherapy drugs and others such as steroids.

The bath can be used to help detoxify the system

by provoking a detoxification reaction, almost by using the age old maxim of *'sweating it out'*. And effectively that is what you hope to achieve by utilising the potential of the skin as *the third kidney.*

A hot bath is one way of achieving this. The temperature range is 100°–107°F (38°–41°C). Hot baths, like cold baths, should only be used for short duration, say a maximum of fifteen minutes for a warm-hot bath, or five minutes maximum for a very hot bath. One should not pour a bath of this temperature and get in suddenly, but start with a warm-tepid bath and gradually increase the heat by adding hot water.

Do always try to shower down or sloosh with cold water before getting out. This closes down the skin pores so that faintness from a sudden drop in blood pressure is less likely.

Note that the time to take a hot bath is in the evening or the end of the day when one does not have to go out again.

After towelling dry and leaving the bathroom, one should take a drink of mineral water, put on nightclothes and retire to bed. One can then expect a perspiration reaction to take place, followed by relaxation and sleepiness. In the morning there may be some noticeable staining of the nightclothes.

An even more potent effect can be obtained by taking an *Epsom Salts Bath.* These famous salts made from hydrated magnesium sulphate, named after the spa town of Epsom with its ancient healing salt spring, are extremely effective in easing pains of the musculoskeletal system and in inducing a detoxification reaction.

To make the bath you take 500 grams of Epsom Salts (available from any chemist) and mix it with almond oil in a basin beside the bath to produce a pleasing wet sand feel.

Draw a hot-tepid bath, so that you will be able to get in with comfort. Stand in the bath and, taking a couple of handfuls of the mixture, rub it over yourself from the neck downwards. Use sweeping movements in the direction of the heart. Do not put on the face or around the genitals.

Put the rest of the Epsom Salts mixture into the bath and stir it with your hands. Then sit down and gently wash the salts off. Then lie down as you increase the temperature to a hot bath. Stay for up to ten minutes.

Having had the bath, shower down quickly with cold or lukewarm water. Take care not to get up too quickly or you might feel faint. Again, have a drink of water, then prepare for bed, making sure that you are wearing nightclothes. The perspiration reaction will take place during the night.

Take an Epsom Salt bath every other day for a week to get a good detoxification reaction.

PRECAUTIONS
• Do listen to the medical advice about when wounds can safely be immersed in water.

• Do make sure that you can get into the bath safely.

• Do make sure that you can comfortably tolerate the bath temperature. Do not run a hot bath and get straight in. Run a warm bath, get in then increase the temperature by adding hot water. Similarly, take care with a cold bath.

• Do use a thermometer to keep the temperature of the bath within the limits suggested.

• Do restrict the time taken in the bath to the suggested times.

Don't
• Do not have a lock on the bathroom door, unless absolutely essential.

• Do not take alcohol or powerful drugs before a bath.

• Do not take a bath after a heavy meal. Two hours should be the minimum, but preferably three hours.

• Do not take a hot bath if there is a history of high blood pressure or heart disease. Have a medical check first.

• Do not use Epsom Salts baths if there has been marked debility and lack of energy.

• Do not use Epsom Salts baths if there is a history of

high blood pressure or heart disease. Check with your health adviser first.

• Do not take hot baths, or Epsom Salts baths if pregnant.

• Do not submit children to hot baths, or Epsom Salts baths.

• Do not get up too quickly after an Epsom Salts bath, or a hot bath. There may be a drop in blood pressure causing unwanted dizziness or even fainting.

• Do not stay longer than the recommended times, particularly with hot baths and detoxification remedies.

• Do not take hot baths if feeling debilitated or low in energy. They will debilitate you more.

• Do not take a hot bath or shower without cool showering down or cooling with cold water. This is necessary to close down the pores.

• Do not take hot baths too early in the day if you have to go out again.

• Do not take cold baths if suffering from intercurrent infections of the respiratory tract.

• Do not take hot baths if there is any neurological impairment of sensation.

• Do not take hot baths if there is any peripheral vascular problem, such as intermittent claudication. This is manifested by pain in the calf muscles on walking short distances.

• Do not take hot baths if there are any vascular complications of Diabetes Melitis, such as leg ulceration.

HELP FOR THE DISABLED

Bathing is something which most able-bodied people take for granted. If the health event has been so severe that one's mobility is significantly impaired then a bath may not be feasible.

If someone has restricted mobility and cannot lie down in the bath, or even sit down, then a bath stool or bath seat may be useful. Bath rails may also help, either fitted to the side of the bath or the front of the bath at the taps end.

Usually an Occupational Therapist can be asked to visit, after referral by the family doctor. They are highly skilled in assessing the needs of people with physical weakness or sensory problems. They can then make recommendations for appropriate fitments to be installed.

The disabled are advised to avoid the extreme temperature therapeutic baths and restrict bathing to medicated baths. If the individual is restricted to a bath seat, high above the water level, then a medicated foot bath with a medicated hand basin will still suffice.

Aromatherapy medicated foot and hand baths are made with half the quantity of essential oils added – 3 or 4 drops will be quite sufficient. In addition, a medicated aromatherapy partial bath (as just described) can be finished off by soaking a towel in the solution and having a wrap around the trunk for up to five minutes. The solution should only be applied warm and should not be left until it is cold.

CHAPTER 8

BREATHE, REST AND MOVE

What is without alternations of rest is not lasting
Ovid

LEARN TO BREATHE

You might think that there is nothing more natural than breathing. Everyone breathes to live. And they do it naturally. There is no learning to be done.

Well, in fact there are two types of breathing – *thoracic*, where the ribcage actually expands and contracts; and *diaphragmatic*, where the ribcage is more or less motionless while the abdomen expands and contracts.

Chest breathers seem to breathe at an average rate of 12–16 full breaths a minute, whereas diaphragmatic breathers only need about 8–10 breaths a minute. If you add that difference up over a whole day it is apparent that there would be a significant 'saving of breath' for the diaphragmatic breathers.

In addition to these two types of breathing there is the point of air entry and exit. That is, there are nose breathers and there are mouth breathers. Quite simply, mouth breathers are by-passing the protective function of the nose. They are depriving themselves of the more measured intake and the filtering process which the nose provides.

In convalescence you really need to maximise your breathing in order to get the maximum effect out of every breath. You need to get the optimum gas transfer of oxygen and carbon dioxide for the least expenditure of energy. The energy saved will be used to boost your recuperation.

There is a branch of yoga called *pranayama,* which is concerned with the simple control of breathing. Controlled breathing will help recovery as well as providing you with a simple means of alleviating the effect of stress. Note the emphasis upon the word 'control', since it means that you are actively seeking to modify the breathing pattern.

Try the following simple exercise and you will be surprised at how relaxed you can make yourself feel.

Begin by sitting in a comfortable position away from noise. Place the hands flat on the abdomen just below the navel, with the fingertips touching.

Now inhale slowly *through the nose*, at the same time pushing the abdomen out so that the fingertips separate. Make sure that you keep the back straight since this will help the lungs fill up with air, and continue to expand the chest and abdomen even after you think that you have inhaled deeply.

Next, raise the shoulders and hold the breath for five seconds. Then slowly exhale *through the nose* as you begin to slowly pull the abdomen in. Let all the air empty by exhaling more deeply than usual. Even then, when you think that you have finished the exhalation, hold your breath for a second or two before starting another slow inhalation *through the nose*.

You should spend five minutes in the morning and five minutes in the evening doing this exercise. If you do, you will gradually change your breathing pattern to become more diaphragmatic. You will start using the nose. You will also certainly start breathing more efficiently.

NOTE: *THIS BREATHING EXERCISE IS USEFUL AFTER SURGERY, CHILDBIRTH AND AFTER MOST ILLNESSES. BUT IF YOU HAVE A SURGICAL WOUND CHECK WITH YOUR HEALTH ADVISER FIRST.*

REST

Ever since the start of the therapeutic revolution of the twentieth century when scientists began discovering the *magic bullets* that we know as steroids, antibiotics, and a host of other genuinely powerful and effective drugs, the focus of Medicine has changed. Whereas at one time the individual had to be treated and nursed through his illness and convalescence, nowadays the illness is the prime aim of treatment. The belief has arisen that the drugs are so powerful that once the acute episode is over recovery will take place swiftly.

While this may be the case with some people, for others it is not so simple. There are all sorts of pressures upon people to get well quickly – financial, occupational and social – and they simply do not take the necessary time to recuperate. The result is that they return to daily activities before their reserves are back to normal. Their function is consequently less than optimal, placing them at greater risk of a relapse, complication or further illness. These sort of factors account for many of the recovery patterns that we covered in Chapter 2. In particular, I believe that they account for the genesis of Chronic Fatigue Syndrome or Myalgic Encephalomyelitis (ME).

This is my first point. After a health event, do not rush back to full activities before you feel able. By this I do not mean that you should argue with your health adviser about the time needed. Indeed, your doctor should be an expert on illness and recovery times. What I mean is that you should accept that advice on recovery time and not try to curtail it so that you risk less than optimum recovery.

My second point is that you should use the methods outlined throughout this book in order to make the recovery curve as close to the ideal as possible. This means taking the time to settle the negative moods (Chapter 3), and allow the natural recovery drive to take place (Chapters 4, 5, 6 and 7).

When resting you should try to disconnect from your usual daily preoccupations. Time should be taken to put the mind into neutral and relax. Read, watch television, enjoy spending time on hobbies and games.

You should take time in the days ahead to learn how to breathe properly. Finally, when appropriate, begin exercising.

MOVEMENT

By movement I mean the whole process of physical movement, not just the process of exercise.

In the old days bed rest was considered a main part of recovery. This is not a good idea for most people, however. The nineteenth century physician and pathologist R.L.K. Virchow realised this when he proposed his famous triad of conditions which predispose an individual to having a thrombosis. These were, damage to the blood vessel walls, stagnation of blood and increased coagulability of the blood. All three of these are more likely after a health event, particularly after prolonged immobilization in bed.

As soon as one can, one should be out of bed and moving around the home. If bed rest is inevitable, through the severity of the illness or because of particular injury or surgery, then it is important to keep the limbs moving every hour. This will tend to counter the effects of *Virchow's triad*.

Broken limbs need some degree of immobilization if they are to heal. This is the reason for using splints and plaster casts. They are simply used to hold the broken ends in close proximity so that bony healing takes place.

Muscle, ligament and joint injuries, however, require movement to help the recovery process. Indeed, they do need active movements from the day of the injury. The help of a physiotherapist or other adviser is of great assistance in this respect.

The very specialised heart muscle needs time to recover after a heart attack or myocardial infarction, so one should take medical advice (which will undoubtedly be given) about when to begin gentle exercises. It is important not to strain the scar tissue of heart muscle.

Surgical operation wounds need to be considered in the same way. The medical advice given post operatively should be strictly adhered to.

Exercises should be started as soon as possible, but this needs to be done sensibly. It is important not to do any strenuous exercise within a week of an acute bacterial or viral illness. Many people may feel that this time is too long, but the truth is that if one tries to exercise the infection away, they risk serious illness. It is not uncommon for such infections to be reactivated in parts of the body that they had not previously affected. Probably the most significant is in the form of a myocarditis, which is an inflammation of the heart. This may create only mild feelings of malaise, but may in reality cover a potentially life-threatening event. People have dropped down dead from unknown myocarditis after exercising too vigorously too soon after an infection.

In starting to exercise one should start very slowly and build up very slowly. Walking is really the finest movement-cum-exercise after most health events. One should be guided by the health adviser about how far they can walk in the first week, then the second week and how long it is expected before one can get back to the normal routine. Again, a physiotherapist or similar adviser can work out a suitable programme for you.

The important thing, however is that movement should begin as early as possible and be gradually built up. You should not force it.

As a rule of thumb, for a young to middle-aged adult, one should use walking as the main movement-cum-exercise for:

• two weeks after an acute infection has been treated
• two weeks after the postnatal period has ended after childbirth
• one month after an operation where the abdomen has been opened
• one month to six weeks after a heart attack without complications
• one month to six weeks after transplantation surgery

AGE AND EXERCISE

It has to be said that people should accept limitations upon their health as they age. This is something which people often find difficult, but it is important.

In a nine-year study of men aged 40–59 years, the

British Heart Foundation followed up 8,000 men in order to assess whether exercise was useful in reducing the risk of heart attacks and strokes. The conclusion was that moderate exercise (a round of golf a week, gardening at the weekend, or a swim) was beneficial in reducing the risk of both heart attacks and strokes. Vigorous exercise, on the other hand was found to reduce further the risk of having a stroke, but increased the risk of having a heart attack.

The message is clear. At about the age of 50 years and onwards, one should not take vigorous exercise, unless one has been used to taking it all one's life. It is a mistake to lead a sedentary life for many years and then suddenly try to get fit. It is much more sensible to follow one's natural constitution. If you have never been really fit, then stick to moderate exercise.

CHAPTER 9

A POCKETFUL OF MAXIMS
– to keep you well

How can we keep our mind and body in the state of harmony which will make it difficult or impossible for disease to attack us....
Edward Bach, *Heal Thyself*

Convalescence doesn't just stop when the individual is over the illness or event and feeling strong enough to return to daily life. There is that all important attitude, that need to stay well and not go back down the same road again.

As a health columnist and practitioner I can think of no better way of advising about this than by drawing upon some old health maxims. In some cases, the wisdom is truly age-old.

*****

....think only of the outlook on life of the one in distress.
Dr Edward Bach

This is one of the most important pieces of advice that I can give. Life is a turbulent process for virtually everyone on the planet. No matter how hard you strive, there will always be unexpected events and happenings which will affect your equanimity. Then again, for no very obvious reason you will find that you wake up one morning and experience a particular negative emotional state. It is like the curtain of doom that descends upon you, the dread of the day ahead, the fear for other people, the sense of guilt, hate, jealousy – all of those emotions which come and dominate your emotional life. And if they persist, then they can reduce your resistance

70

and before you know it you are facing another health event.

The beauty of the Bach Flower Remedies is that they can rapidly correct and remove these negative mental states. By focusing upon how you feel in the morning, by pinpointing any negative feelings and taking the appropriate remedy at breakfast you can get the day off to a good start.

Most people will find that their particular negative states can be dealt with by about six of the remedies. Thus, a small investment can repay itself many times over in terms of improved health.

*****

Breakfast like a king, lunch like a prince, supper like a pauper.
Old Proverb

This has to do with sensible eating. Most people's eating patterns have more to do with social conditioning than actual needs. We are programmed by society to have three square meals a day. More than that, we are programmed to have a little breakfast, a snack for lunch, then a large evening meal. This is absolutely the wrong way round.

A little thought will reveal that the time when you need the most calories is in the morning. You should take the fuel on board in order to work it off throughout the day. Hence the above maxim. Having the bulk of the calories after the day's work has been performed is of little sense, since the surplus to required calories will be stored as body fat. In addition, the circulating fat creates the right conditions for the laying down of fat in blood vessels, the very origin of arteriosclerosis.

There is also good scientific evidence which shows that the three square meals idea is wrong. Human beings have the digestive tracts of grazing animals rather than that of guzzlers. That means that we are better suited to having many small meals more frequently. It has been shown that if one takes the

71

same calorific intake of food scattered over say six to eight small meals rather than three, then the levels of blood glucose, cholesterol and insulin remain steady and at a more controlled level.

Do therefore try to get the balance of your diet more in line with the above maxim. Or better still, try eating small and often.

*****

An apple a day keeps the doctor away.
Old Proverb

The concept here is that one should eat fruit (and nuts) every day. At least two pieces. It is good for the anti-oxidants, vitamins, minerals and fibre (see Chapter 5).

*****

Light supper makes long life
Medieval Proverb

This follows on from the observation that those who sleep well tend to enjoy long and good health. Certainly, overloading the digestion at night can hinder sleep.This was also observed in Roman times:

From a great supper comes a great pain; that you may sleep lightly sup lightly
Latin Proverb

*****

Rest after lunch; after supper walk
Maxim of the Medical School of Salerno (12th Century)

This is an incredibly intuitive observation. Physio-logically, we are at our lowest ebb in the early afternoon. This is why the concept of the siesta makes such good sense. Many of our hormones have an M-shaped distribution, being at peak levels in the early day and in the evening.

Exercise in the early afternoon is not always the best time. You are far better to wait until the late afternoon or early evening after the last meal.

*****

Exercise and temperance can preserve something of our early strength even in old age
Cicero

Here we have a caution not to become too sedentary as we age. Similarly, one should avoid taking too many stimulants into our systems.

*****

Finally, my personal favourite which really says it all:

Moderation in all things is the best of rules
Plautus

INDEX